YOUR GUIDE TO A SUITABLE CONTRACEPTIVE METHOD

BY

KIBOKO FRANÇOISE MACHOZI

www.savelife.co.za

CONTENTS

INTRODUCTION

To have a child is a responsibility that involves love, attention, time, and money. A couple must be prepared before both partners may decide to have a child. There are people who abuse their own children; others conceive children, deliver them properly, and give them up or undergo an abortion just because they were not ready to have children, but the truth is that abortion is killing, despite the reason. It is better to give up a baby after delivery than to abuse him or her or have an abortion, and it is much better to prevent getting pregnant than to give up a child.

This is the reason that motivated me to write this book, which tells you about the contraceptive methods that will help you prevent unplanned pregnancies, as they can sometimes lead to child abuse and abortion, which is a crime.

1. ANATOMY OF A FEMALE REPRODUCTIVE SYSTEM

The female reproductive system is subdivided into two different parts: the internal and the external part (or vulva).

1. 1. INTERNAL FEMALE REPRODUCTIVE SYSTEM

1. UTERUS

The uterus is a median, pear-shaped, hollow, muscular, and elastic organ in which the fertilized ovum becomes an embryo, a fetus, and, later, a baby. It is situated in the pelvis between the bladder at the front and the rectum at the back side.

It is composed of two parts: the body (the upper part) and the cervix (lower part), which opens into the vagina below and into the uterine cavity above.

The uterus has three layers:

- the endometrium or inner layer of the uterus cavity, on which a fertilized ovum fixes itself

(NB: Damage to the endometrium may cause adhesion and fibrosis, which are not favorable for the fixation of a fertilized ovum.)

- the myometrium or uterus muscles
- the perimetrium or uterus envelope

The uterus weighs between fifty and seventy grams. It measures plus minus seven and half centimeters in length.[i]

2. VAGINA

The vagina is an elastic and muscular canal going from the lower part of the uterus (cervix) to the vulva. It measures approximately nine centimeters in length and six to seven and half centimeters in diameter.

Its roles consist of allowing intercourse, the passage of sperm to the uterus, the passage of menstruations to the vulva, and the passage of a child during birth.

The vagina allows the examination of the uterine cervix. It also allows different maneuvers to be performed in the uterus.

Bartholin glands or greater vestibular glands are two mucoid-secreting glands located in the lower part of the vagina, one at the left side and the other at the right. These glands produce a mucoid substance, which makes the vagina smooth and wet to avoid dryness and irritation.[ii]

3. FALLOPIAN TUBES

Fallopian tubes are two canals situated on both the left and the right sides of the upper lateral part of the uterus body. Each fallopian tube measures seven to fourteen centimeters in length. Fallopian tubes connect the uterus to the ovaries, allowing the passage of both spermatozoids from the uterus and ovum from the ovary to meet each other inside it. Fallopian tubes also allow the passage of a fertilized egg to the uterus.

Cilia and fluids found inside the fallopian tubes allow an ovum and a fertilized egg to move smoothly toward the uterus.

A fallopian tube has four parts:

- isthmus which is a narrower part that links to the cavity of the uterus
- ampulla (the portion where a spermatozoid meets an ovum)
- infundibulum which is the third part of a Fallopian tube that is situated between the ampoulla and the fimbria
- fimbria which is the last part of the fallopian tube in the direction of the ovary and which captures the egg once it is delivered by the ovary.

A fertilized egg takes seven days (from the ampulla) before it reaches the uterus.

A fallopian tube has three layers:

- Mucosa is the internal layer, which has ciliated cells.

- Muscularis (muscle) is the middle layer of a fallopian tube, which has nerves and allows motion.
- Serosa is the external layer or envelope of a fallopian tube.[iii]

4. OVARIES

Ovaries are oval organs situated at the end of each fallopian tube. They deliver an ovum once a month and produce hormones.[iv]

1. 2. THE EXTERNAL FEMALE REPRODUCTIVE SYSTEM

1. Labium majus are two lateral structures that cover and protect the external female reproductive system from germs.
They have glands that produce sweat and oil to protect the external female reproductive system from dryness and irritation.

2. Labium minus are folds of mucous membrane located at the left and right sides of the vaginal entrance. They have their origins in the lower

part of the clitoris. They cover and protect the vaginal entrance from germs.

3. The clitoris is an erectile organ found in the anterior part of the vulva.

4. The vaginal orifice is a small hole situated in the middle posterior part of the vulva under the

two labium minus, between the orifices of both the urethra and the anus at the back side.[v]

2. FEMALE HORMONES

Hormones are chemical substances produced by glands. They move inside the body through the bloodstream and regulate the functions of others organs. Hormones work like messengers between different organs inside a human body.

Sex glands produce hormones during fetal development, but they become inactive during childhood.

At birth, a baby girl has 450,000 eggs in her ovaries. Each of them is found in an envelope called a follicle. At puberty, a teenager's body starts to produce hormones that mature her eggs.

Female hormones are produced by ovaries. They produce estrogen, progesterone, and much more.

In this section we will focus on estrogen and progesterone. Estrogen builds up the uterine lining, thickens the vaginal lining, stimulates the breast tissue, promotes the building of bones, and protects the cardiovascular system.[vi]

Progesterone prepares the uterine lining to bear the fertilized ovum, increases sexual desire, increases energy, and develops muscles.

3. MENSTRUAL CYCLE

The hypothalamus is a gland in a human being's brain controlling the menstrual cycle. It releases a chemical called "follicles stimulating hormones regulating factor," or FSH-RF, to give information to the pituitary (the second gland in the brain), so it may release FSH in the blood stream. FSH increases blood supply in ovaries and promotes the maturation of follicles in the ovaries.

The maturing follicle releases another hormone called estrogen, which thickens the uterus lining and prepares it to bear a child. Also, it changes the appearance of the cervical mucus, which becomes slippery and transparent like a raw egg.

High levels of estrogen decrease the basal temperature (vaginal temperature) and stimulate the hypothalamus to produce another chemical called "leutenizing hormones regulating factor" (LH-RF), which makes the pituitary gland release the leutenizing hormone (LH). This hormone makes the most mature follicle burst and release the egg. This process is called ovulation.

Before ovulation, the blood supply in the ovaries increases; there is a contraction of ligaments, which allows the ovaries to be closer to the fallopian tubes and easily transfer the egg from the ovary to the fallopian tube once it is released.

The cervix releases stretchy, clear mucus, which allows the easy passage of spermatozoid to meet the egg inside the fallopian tube. Inside the fallopian tube, the egg movement is made possible by cilia.

From ovulation to menstruation, the follicle that released an ovum is called a corpus luteum or "yellow body" because of its color. This produces estrogen and a large amount of progesterone for the maintenance of the pregnancy. If there is no fertilization, the yellow body becomes white, and it is called corpus albicans.

Progesterone increases basal temperature; it makes the glands of the uterus lining produce mucous, which covers the internal part of the uterus (endometrium). If there is no fertilization, the uterus lining will be destroyed and convert into menstruations.[vii]

MENSTRUATIONS OR MENSES

This is a physiologic bloody discharge that comes from the uterus and occurs every month. It is a common process for women from puberty to menopause.

THE LENGTH OF YOUR MENSTRUAL CYCLE

A menstrual cycle is a period that starts from the first day of your last menstruation period until the day of your next menstruation.

How do you know the length of your menstrual cycle?

To know the length of your cycle, you have to write down (on a personal calendar) the first day of your menstruations, and, after six to twelve months, you calculate the number of days between two menstruation periods.

For example

In January, you had your menstruation on the fourteenth.

In February, you had your menstruation on the seventeenth.

In March, you had your menstruation on the seventeenth.

In April, you had your menstruation on the sixteenth.

In May, you had your menstruation on the twentieth.

In June, you had your menstruation on the twenty-second.

In July, you had your menstruation on the twenty-first.

In August, you had your menstruation on the seventeenth.

In September, you had your menstruation on the fourteenth.

In October, you had your menstruation on the fourteenth.

In November, you had your menstruation on the fifteenth.

In December, you had your menstruation on the fourteenth.

From January to February, there were thirty-five days before you menstruated.

From February to March, there were twenty-nine days before you menstruated.

From March to April, there were thirty-one days before you menstruated.

From April to May, there were thirty-five days before you menstruated.

From May to June, there were thirty-four days before you menstruated.

From June to July, there were thirty days before you menstruated.

From July to August, there were twenty-eight days before you menstruated.

From August to September, there were twenty-nine days before you menstruated.

From September to October, there were thirty-one days before you menstruated.

From October to November, there were thirty-three days before you menstruated.
From November to December, there were thirty days before you menstruated.

Your longest cycle has thirty-five days, and your shortest cycle has twenty-eight days.
The average cycle =
$$\frac{\text{your longest cycle} + \text{your shortest cycle}}{2}$$
35+28=63/2=31.5=32

ESTIMATION OF THE DATE OF YOUR NEXT MENSTRUATIONS

To estimate the day of your next menstruation, you have to know the length of your cycle, and, from there, you count down on a calendar the average number of days of your cycle, starting from the first day of your last menstruation forward and find out the approximate day of your next menstruation.

For example

You had your last menstruation on January 3.
Your cycle has approximately thirty-two days.

Your next menstruation will be around February 3.

OVULATION

Ovulation is the liberation of an ovum by an ovary. This occurs once during a menstrual cycle.

To estimate the day of your ovulation, you first have to estimate the date of your next menstruation; from there, on the calendar count backward fourteen days toward the last menstruation, and the fifteenth day is your estimated day of ovulation.

This is the right time to have sex or to avoid it, depending on whether or not you want to get pregnant.

Menstruations always happen fourteen days after ovulation.

NB: Actually, there are specific tests that help you find out exactly when you will be ovulating by checking the urine or the saliva. Those tests may predict your ovulation day up to seven days beforehand.

OULATION SIGNS

- Increase in the amount and texture of cervical mucus

(It stretches and becomes slippery and clear like a raw egg because of the sharp rise in estrogen.)

- Discomfort in the lower part of the abdomen

(This pain is interpreted as tension caused by a follicle that is about to burst.)

- Slight bleeding in the middle of the cycle

- Change in position and firmness of the cervix

- Increased sexual desire

- Increased breast sensitivity

A sharp rise in body temperature is proof that you ovulated the day before.

After ovulation, the yellow body starts to produce progesterone, which increases the woman's body temperature.

A vaginal smear done during the first part of the cycle or follicular is clear, but the one done during the second part of the cycle or luteal is dirty.

An endometrium biopsy performed between the twenty-first and the twenty-fifth day of the cycle shows signs of ovulation.

A coelioscopy done in the middle of the cycle shows a mature follicle ready to rupture or already ruptured and transformed into a yellow body.

METHODS USED TO LOCATE THE APPROXIMATE TIME OF OVULATION

The menstrual cycle has two different phases:
The first phase or estrogenic phase—Its length may change due to different reasons, e.g., emotion, stress, diseases, weather, and much more.

The length of the second phase is constant and does not change due to any circumstance. The length is fourteen days. Once a woman ovulates, she has to count fourteen days before she will see her menstruations.

Ovulation calendar:

With this method, a woman will have to estimate the date of her next menstruation; from there, she will count backward fourteen days and can evaluate approximately the date on which she will be ovulating. To prevent a pregnancy, she should avoid sexual intercourse during this period, or she may use any barrier method.

You may also calculate your fertile period by the following method:

Calculate and find out your longest and your shortest cycle.
From your shortest cycle, count backward eighteen days, starting with the last day to find out the first day of the fertile period of your current cycle.

From your longest cycle, count backward eleven days starting with the last day, to find out the last day of the fertile period of the current cycle. The days in between are your fertile period.

For an illustration: your longest cycle counts thirty-five days and your shortest twenty-nine.

Your last menstruations were on the eighteen July 2013.

On a calendar, considering your shortest cycle, your next menstruations may be on the fifteen of August. From this date, you count backward eighteen days, to find out the first day of the fertile period, it will be the twenty-nine of July.

Considering your longest cycle, your next menstruation may be on the twenty-first of August 2013. Starting with this date, you count backward eleven days to determine the last day of your July fertile period, it will be the eleven of August.

Your July fertile period goes from the twenty-nine July to the eleven of August 2013. You will have to abstain during this period of time in order to prevent pregnancy.

Evaluation of cervical mucus texture:

To avoid the likelihood of pregnancy, a woman will have to check and evaluate the texture, appearance, and color of her cervical mucus every morning, and she should not have sexual intercourse once the texture of the cervical mucus increases and becomes slippery.

Measure of basal temperature:

To avoid the likelihood of pregnancy, a woman should check her vaginal temperature using a digital basal thermometer every morning. A day before ovulation, the temperature will decrease; once the temperature rises, the woman knows that she ovulated the day before. She should avoid sex during this period.

Urine-based ovulation test:

This test is accurate and helps a woman know the exact day she ovulates.

Fertility monitor:

This is a small machine that uses saliva to check the ovulation. This machine may predict ovulation up to seven days before by checking the level of progesterone, the level of estrogen, or both.

NB: An ovum may only live for twenty-four, hours while a spermatozoid may live up to five days. This means a woman may still become pregnant from sexual intercourse she had five days before ovulation and a day after ovulation.[viii]

4. PREGNANCY

Pregnancy is the state of a female after conception and until the termination of the gestation.[1]

Conception: fertilization of an ovum by a spermatozoid
Gestation: the fact of bearing a fertilized ovum

---

[1]*Stedman's Medical Dictionary for the Health Professions and*

5. CONTRACEPTIVE METHODS

Contraceptive methods are different techniques used with the purpose of controlling fertility and the prevention of conception or impregnation.[2] This can be temporary or permanent.

Contraceptives are used for different reasons:

-Personal reasons

- To postpone the possibility of having another child while the couple has a baby
- Refusal to bear children
- Avoidance of being tempted to have an abortion

-Medical reasons

- When pregnancy can compromise the life of the mother (women suffering from heart disease)
- or when the baby has a risk of being contaminated by the sick mother (e.g., in

---

[2] Ibid., page

- the case of an HIV-positive mother with a high viral load)

-Socioeconomic reasons

- When a couple does not have enough of an income to fulfill the baby's needs

There are different contraceptive methods.

5. 1. NATURAL METHODS

ABSTINENCE

Abstinence can be partial or total.

-Total abstinence:

We talk about total abstinence when a person totally avoids sex.

-Partial abstinence:

We talk about partial abstinence when a couple avoids having sex during a fertile period.

In this category of contraception, the couple focuses on checking the ovulation period and avoids sex during this specific time. This method requires sufficient knowledge of ovulation signs.

Both of these methods have a high percentage of failure.

BREASTFEEDING

Breastfeeding stimulates the pituitary gland to produce more prolactin and oxytocin. Prolactin promotes the change of blood into breast milk, and oxytocin pushes out breast milk. The contraceptive effect of breastfeeding is not well understood, but the presence of prolactin inhibits the secretion of LH (a hormone that induces ovulation).

For breastfeeding to be effective as a contraceptive method, there are conditions to be met:

- The woman must only give breast milk to her baby, not artificial milk.
- The baby must be breastfed on demand, regularly and without delay.
- The mother must combine breastfeeding with a contraceptive method that is compatible with breastfeeding once she sees her menstruations.

5. 2. ARTIFICIAL METHODS

1. BARRIER METHODS

Mechanical and chemical methods:

1. 1. MECHANICAL METHODS:

This is a mechanical device that blocks the passage of sperm to a woman's uterus. In this group we find:
Male and female condoms
Vaginal sponge
Diaphragm
Cervical cap

Male condoms

This is a tube-like latex covering that a male puts on his penis once he has an erection and removes after sexual intercourse. It must only be used once. This method protects from pregnancy and from sexually transmissible diseases.

Vaginal sponge

It is a sponge containing dry spermicidal foam that dissolves once it absorbs vaginal secretions or sperm. This sponge is put in the vagina and acts in three major ways:

- Obstructing the cervix and forbidding spermatozoid penetration
- Absorbing sperm
- Releasing spermicides

A vaginal contraceptive sponge must be put in the vagina less than two hours from the time it is removed from its original wrapper, fifteen minutes before intercourse, and must stay in the vagina eight hours after the last ejaculation. It may be used over twenty-four hours from the time it was put in the vagina but must be thrown away once it is removed.

Always check the expiration date before using a vaginal contraceptive sponge as it is no longer effective afterward.[ix]

Diaphragm contraceptive

This is a cervical barrier made with latex or silicone deposited in the vagina to block spermatozoids passing toward the womb.
For proper security, a spermicidal cream or gel must be applied on the device.

This device may stay in the vagina for twenty-four hours and may be used several times within the twenty-four hours. Once a diaphragm has been removed from the vagina, it must be washed properly, dried, and well-kept as it may be used several times.

A diaphragm must be prescribed by a healthcare professional after a complete gynecologic examination, which will determine the size of the device. A latex diaphragm must be renewed every two years, but a silicone one may last up to ten years.
NB: Avoid using oily lubricants as they may easily destroy the latex.[x]

Cervical caps

This is a sort of a cover put on the cervix to prevent the penetration of spermatozoids. For proper protection, a spermicidal cream or gel must be applied.

A cap may stay on the cervix for up to seventy-two hours from the time of insertion, and, it must stay on the cervix eight hours after the last ejaculation.

After a cap has been removed from the vagina, it must be properly washed with soap, dried, and well-kept as it may be used several times, but it must be renewed every two years. A cap must be prescribed by a healthcare professional after a complete gynecological examination, which will determine the size of the device.[xi]

1. 2. CHEMICAL METHODS

These include spermicidal gel, foam, cream, and tablets. Chemical contraceptives are put in the vagina before intercourse in order to kill spermatozoids before they reach the uterus.

2. HORMONAL METHODS

Hormonal contraceptives must be prescribed after a complete gynecologic examination to determine the physical conditions and tendencies of a woman, as there are women with high levels of progesterone. They must not use contraceptives that have high levels of progesterone but can use those with high levels of estrogen. There are also women with high levels of estrogen; they must not use contraceptives with high levels of estrogen but can use those with high levels of progesterone to equilibrate their hormonal secretions.

There are pills, injections, subcutaneous implants, patches, vaginal rings and Intra Uterine System. All of these contain synthetic hormones that inhibit LH secretion and inhibit ovulation as well. They are used for different purposes, which may be to:
- prevent pregnancy
- regulate menstruation
- prevent ovulation pain
- prevent menstruation pain
- prevent heavy flow and avoid anemia
- equilibrate hormonal secretion

Medicine interaction

Some medications may decrease the efficacy of hormonal contraceptives:
Rifampicin
Rifabutin
Phenytoin
Tegretol
Phenobarbital
Primidone

2. 1. ORAL CONTRACEPTIVES

There are two different kinds: *estroprogestatives* and mini pills.

Estroprogestatives: These pills are composed of both estrogen and progestin. Among them we have different groups:

1. *Monophasic* pills: they have a constant dose of estrogen and a lower dose of progestin for twenty-one days.
E.g.: Ovral, Nordette, Yasmin, Liette, Adco-Fem-35, Diane-35, Cilest, Levlitte, Mircette, Loestrin fe

2. *Biphasic* pills: the hormone (estrogen and progestin) doses are not constant for the whole cycle; an adjustment is made once in the middle of the cycle.
E.g.: Biphasil, Evra, Jenest

3. Triphasic estrogen and progesterone: an adjustment is made twice within twenty-one days.
E.g.: Triphasil, Triodene ED, Trinovum, Ortho-Novum

4. Morning-after pill: this is a pill with a higher dose of estrogen. This pill must be taken up to 120 hours after unprotected sex.
NB: This pill acts as a contraceptive method only if it is taken before ovulation or before a spermatozoid may enter an ovum, otherwise it will be acting as an abortive method. **It prevents the fixation of the fertilized egg in the uterus. It is not a contraceptive but an abortive method.**

2. Mini pills or progestin-only pills: just like their name implies, these pills have only one hormone, which is progesterone. They are useful

for women who, for one reason or another, cannot take synthetic estrogen.
E.g.: Microval, Micro-Novum, Norlevo, Levonorgestrel, Norithindone

Advantages of oral contraceptives:

Oral contraceptives give the possibility of postponing the next menstruation period.
With oral contraceptives, you can predict the date of the next menstruations. You can decide which day of the week you do not want to menstruate by taking your first tablet on that specific day.
Oral contraceptives:
Regulate menses
Eliminate menstruation pain
Solve uterine bleeding problems
Treat the skin
Decrease the risk of ovarian and endometrium cancer

Disadvantages of oral contraceptives:

Oral contraceptives:
Delay the return of fertility (It can take two to three months for fertility to restart.)

Cause hypertension
Lead to blood clots
Cause nausea
Have a high percentage of failure because of forgetfulness

NB: Researchers are learning about a birth control pill that will not use hormonal content but the zp3 protein found on female eggs called pellucid. They are trying to make a product that will fix itself to that specific protein and prevent the formation of pellucid. By doing so, spermatozoids will not gain entry into the female egg.

Actually, there is a male birth control pill that is made with a chemical called JQ1 that temporarily stops the BRDT (protein located in testicles that promotes the production of spermatozoids) from producing spermatozoids. This product does not have side effects and its effect is reversible.

2. 2. INJECTABLE CONTRACEPTIVES

These contraceptives are used as temporary methods. They are made with a progestational compound only. Actually, there are only two:

1. Noristerate or norethindrone enanthate or net en:
   This product must be given every two months.
2. Depo-provera or medroxy progesterone acetate:
   This product must be given every
   three months.

For good results, injectable contraceptives must be given through intramuscular injection. The first injection must be given between the first and the fifth day of menses or immediately after menses. After giving birth, the injection must be given six weeks later or seven days after a miscarriage or abortion.

These injections must be done on the appointed day or at least four days before or after the appointed date.

Advantages of injectable contraceptives:

- The rate of failure is less than 1 percent.
- The effectiveness starts from twenty-four hours after the injection.
- Injectable contraceptives do not affect breastfeeding.
- Injectable contraceptives do not have estrogen and do not affect blood pressure.
- Injectable contraceptives do not interfere with intercourse.
- Injectable contraceptives do not cause nausea.
- They decrease the risk of endometrial cancer.
- They decrease the risk of benign breast disease.
- They prevent pelvic inflammatory disease.

Disadvantages:

- Menses irregularity
- No possibility of postponing menstruations or predicting the next menstruation period

- Delay the return of fertility (It can take four to five months for fertility to become normal.)
- Loss of bone mass by decreasing calcium concentration in bones
- Heavy bleeding
- Mood swings
- Loss of hair
- Decrease or increase of facial or body hair
- Rash
- Weight increase
- Tenderness of breasts
- Testosterone suppression, which decreases libido
- Headaches
- Nervousness
- Increases the risk of breast and uterine cancers
- Increases the risk of blood clots in lungs and legs
- Jaundice
- Allergic reaction
- Infertility

Women with liver disease, blood clot history, and strokes should avoid injectable contraceptives. Injectable contraceptives must not be given to girls under the age of sixteen because of bone decalcification. Injectable contraceptives must be avoided if the woman plans to conceive in the next year.

2. 3. IMPLANTS

This is a thin rod containing etonorgestrel.
It is inserted in the left upper arm eight to ten centimeters above the elbow. From under the skin, it releases a steady amount of etonorgestrel into the bloodstream. The hormones reach your ovaries and prevent ovulation. It makes changes to the uterus lining and cervix. It can work for three years (e.g., implant etonogestrel).

It must be inserted between the first and the fifth day of menses; it can be put in after giving birth as well and removed three to four years later.

Side effects:

Implants do not lead to cancer, but the product in it may increase the risk of breast cancer.

Advantages:

Unlike injection, implants can be removed at any time.

Disadvantages:

Vaginal bleeding
Spots/acne
Weight increase
Depression
Dizziness
Low sexual desire
Headaches

2.4.CONTRACEPTIVE PATCH

It is an estro-progestative compound on an adhesive plastic/bandage applied to the lower abdomen, waist, which steadily releases a small amount of hormones.

NB: A patch must never be applied onto the breast.

2. 5. VAGINAL RINGS

These are soft, flexible pieces of plastic that contain synthetic hormones that must be progressively absorbed inside the vagina. The hormonal content within them prevents ovulation, changes the uterus lining, and thickens cervical mucus.

The ring is inserted inside the vagina for three weeks, removed at the fourth week, and will be replaced at the end of the fourth week.

Advantages:

It can be removed at any time.

Side effects:

Nausea
Headaches
Dizziness
Fatigue
Breast tenderness
Loss of appetite
Weight gain

Precaution:

Vaginal rings should not be put inside women who smoke, women with a history of uterus or breast cancer, women with a history of hypertension, heart attack, or blood clots, women with diabetes mellitus, or women with liver disease, vaginal bleeding, or allergies.

2.6. INTRAUTERINE SYSTEM

It is a T-shaped device containing progesterone and releasing it steadily on a regular basis. This device may be effective for up to five years from the time it has been inserted in the uterus.

How do hormonal contraceptives work?

Hormonal contraceptives inhibit the secretion of LH by the pituitary gland and prohibit the liberation of an ovum by the follicle (ovulation). They thicken the uterus lining and prevent the fixation of the fertilized egg on the endometrium. They also thicken cervical mucus and prohibit the penetration of spermatozoids.

Advantages of hormonal contraceptives:

Hormonal contraceptives decrease menstrual cramps, decrease bleeding, improve anemia, prevent ectopic pregnancy, control fertility, and prevent abortion.[xii]

3. SURGICAL METHODS

3. 1. TUBAL LIGATION

This is a surgical female contraceptive method that involves the closure of fallopian tubes (tubes that connect ovaries to the uterus and where an ovum is fertilized by a spermatozoid).

3. 2. VASECTOMY

This is a surgical male contraceptive method that involves the cutting of small tubes that are canals used by sperm carrying spermatozoids from testicles to the semen (*vas deferens*).

Advantages of surgical methods:

Successful

Disadvantages:

In most cases, the process is irreversible.
Post-surgery pain
Post-surgery infection is possible.
Chronic pain may occur in some few cases.

CONCLUSION

If there is a way to prevent unwanted pregnancy, it is better to do so. Do not wait for the worst case and give excuses. This will not help you, but it may lead you to some other mistakes that may have more consequences than the previous one. As you discovered in this book, there are several contraceptive methods that may help you prevent unplanned pregnancies.

[i] Linda, et al, 2012, "Uterus," MedlinePlus medical encyclopedia, image found at www.nlm.nih.gov/../19263.htm
[ii] "Vagina" found at www.wikipedia.org/wiki/vagina
[iii] Definition of fallopian tube found at www.medterms.com/script/main/ art.as...
Fallopian tube found at www.wikipedia.org/wiki/Fallopiantube
Fallopian tube, *Encyclopaedia Britannica*, found at www.britanica.com

[iv] Ovarian disorders, MedlinePlus, found at www.nlh.nih.gov/MedlinePlus/Ovarian...
[v] Body basics, female reproductive system: about human reproduction, found at www.kidshealth.org>Kids health>Parents>General health

[vi] Follicule ovarian, www.wikipedia.org/wiki/../follicule_ovarian
Cancer info, En savoir plus sur les hormones feminines, found at www.e.cancer.fr>accueil>info patient>Les cancers>cancer du sein>hormonotherapy
Eureka santé, Les hormones feminines et le cycle menstrual, Que faire en cas d'oublie de la pillule? J'ai oublie ma pillule, www.eurekasante.fr>Accueil>Maladies>Sexualite et contraception
Hypothalamus found at www.wikipedia.org/wiki/hypothalamus
Hypophyse, Futura-sante,www.futura-sciences.com/fr/definition...
Dr Aly Abbara, 2012, "Oestrogenes," www.aly-abbara.com/../oestrogenes.html
Progesterone, www.wikipedia.org/wiki/progest%25C3%...

[vii] Cycle et ovulation, www.doctissimo.fr/htm/sexualite/education
Cancer info, En savoir plus sur les hormones feminines, found at www.e.cancer.fr>accueil>info patient>Les cancers>cancer du sein>hormonotherapy.
Eureka santé, Les hormones feminines et le cycle menstrual, Que faire en cas d'oublie de la pillule? J'ai oublie ma pillule, www.eurekasante.fr>Accueil>Maladies>Sexualite et contraception
Hypothalamus found at www.wikipedia.org/wiki/hypothalamus

Hypophyse, Futura-sante,www.futura-sciences.com/fr/definition...
Dr Aly Abbara, 2012, Oestrogenes, www.aly-abbara.com/../oestrogenes.html
Progesterone, www.wikipedia.org/wiki/progest%25C3%...

[viii] Best fertility monitor, www.bestfertility monitor.com/

[ix] Planned Parenthood, birth control sponge (Today Sponge), found at www.walgreens.com>Home>Shop.
Vaginal sponge and spermicides, www.nlm.nih.gov/../004003.htm
[x] Diaphragm (contraceptive), www.wikipedia.org/wiki/Diaphragm_Co...
[xi] Cervical cap (fem cap), found at www.plannedparenthood.org/Health.to...
[xiixii] Patient information, hormonal method of birth control (beyond the basics) found at www.uptodate.com/Content/Hormonal...
Hormonal method of birth control (cont.) found at www.medicinenet.com/../article.htm
Contraception guide found at www.nhs.uk/conditions/contraception...